AN EASY-READ COMMUNITY BOOK

WHO KEEPS US HEALTHY?

BY CAROLINE ARNOLD

PHOTOGRAPHS BY CAROLE BERTOL

Franklin Watts
New York/London/Toronto/Sydney
1982

Special thanks are due the following individuals and organizations whose cooperation made the photographs possible:

Buchanan County Dept. of Health and Welfare; Pammy Lee and Thomas Campbell; Eva Carrigher; The Gingerbread House; Hudson Guild Fulton Senior Center; B. Ivanovich; Dr. Amy Kapatkin; Mrs. F.R. Kort; Debbie Martie; Kathy Merrick; Alice McVicker; Methodist Medical Center; Janet Moser; Mary Noone; North Shore Animal League; NYC Dept. for the Aging-Cornell Medical College Hypertension Care Program; Dr. Helen Nguyen; Oak Cliff Medical and Surgical Hospital; Brigid Pace; Elaine Quigley; Dr. Morton Samet; Peggy Schaag; Anna Schoepf; Jennifer and Jessica Scott; Leonard Shaykin; Dr. Warren A. Shoecraft; Leslie Speiser; Universal Health Services, Inc.; West Side Branch YMCA of Greater New York.

Photographs on page 23 courtesy of International Center for the Disabled; on pages 27 and 31 by Paul Conklin from Monkmeyer Press Photo Service

R.L. 2.4 Spache Revised Formula

Library of Congress Cataloging in Publication Data

Arnold, Caroline.
Who keeps us healthy?

(An Easy-read community book)
Includes index.
Summary: Briefly introduces and explains the work of various health care professionals and examines programs which promote publich health.
1.Medical personnel—Juvenile literature. 2. Community health services—Juvenile literature. [1. Medical personnel. 2. Occupations. 3. Public health]
I. Bertol, Carole, ill. II. Title. III. Series.
R690.A7 1982   610.69   82-8545
ISBN 0-531-04440-8   AACR2

Text copyright © 1982 by Caroline Arnold
Illustrations copyright © 1982 by Franklin Watts, Inc.
All rights reserved
Printed in the United States of America
6 5 4 3 2 1

CONTENTS

Health Care People 6
Places Where Health Care People Work 15
Communities Help People Stay Healthy 24

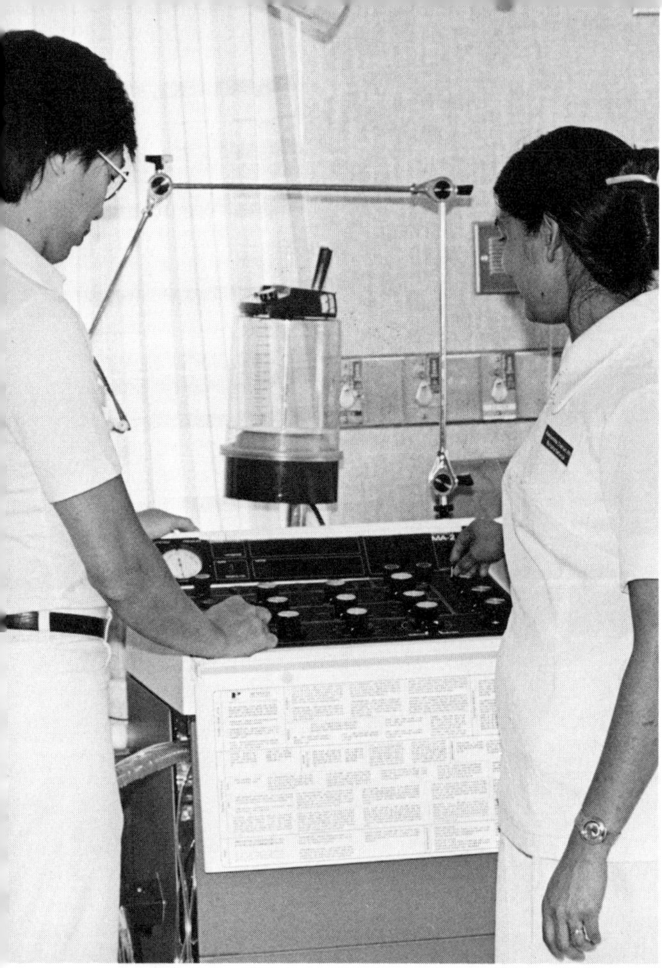

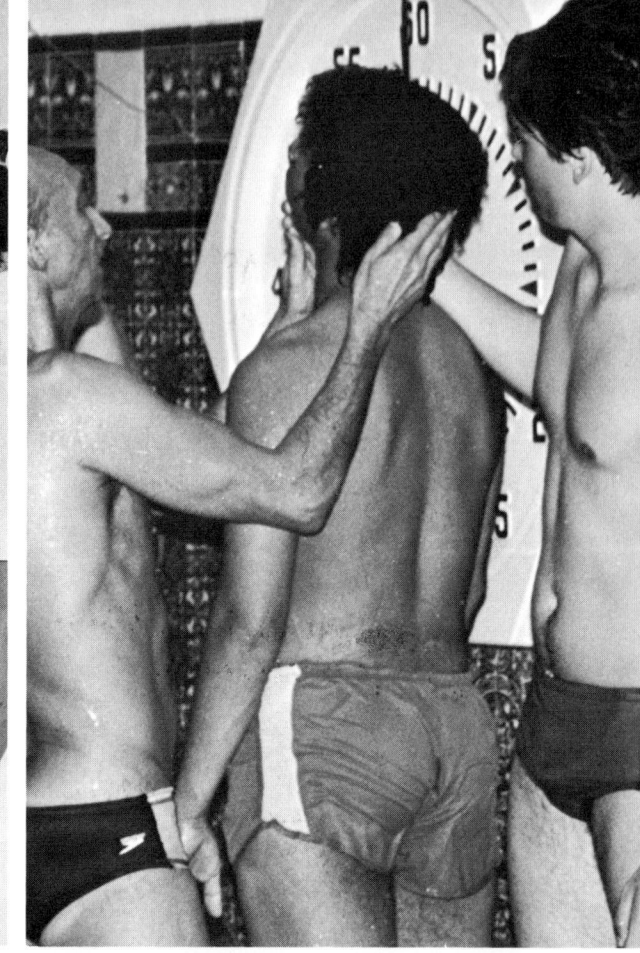
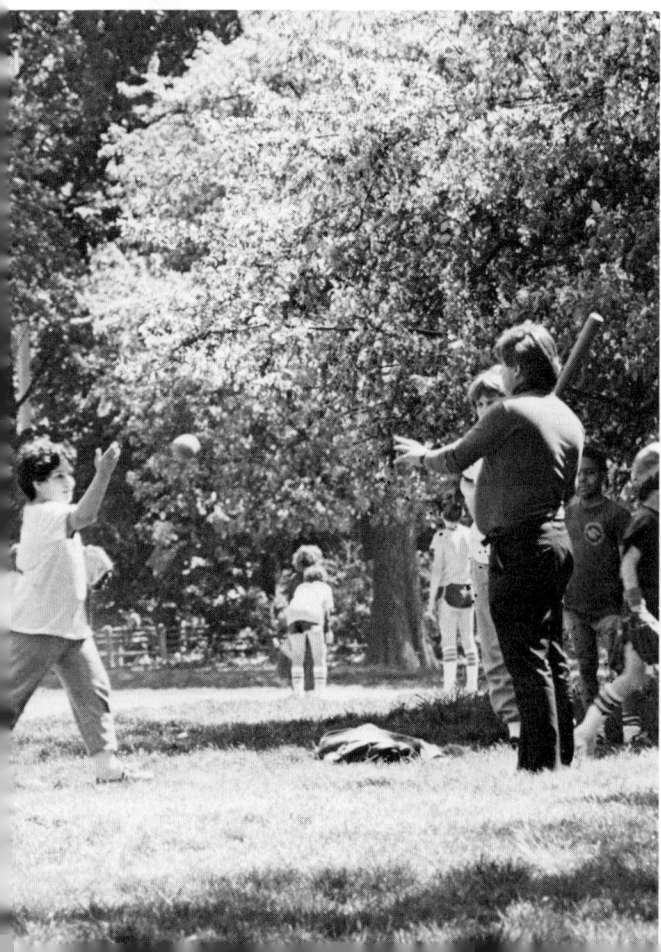
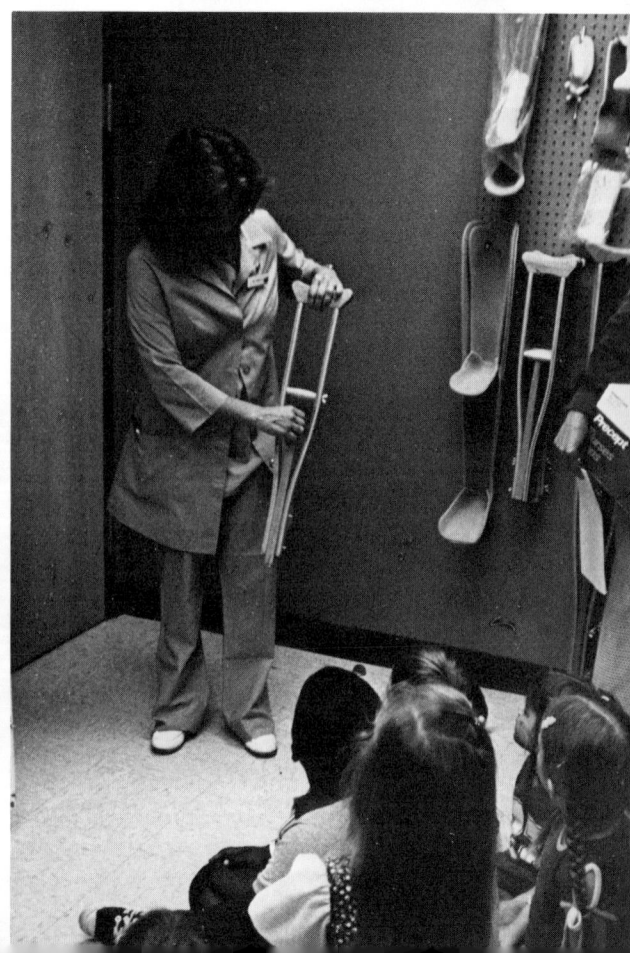

Good health is important for all of us. When we feel well we can work and play at our best.

Do you eat good foods each day?

Do you exercise every day?

Do you get enough sleep each night?

All these things help people stay healthy.

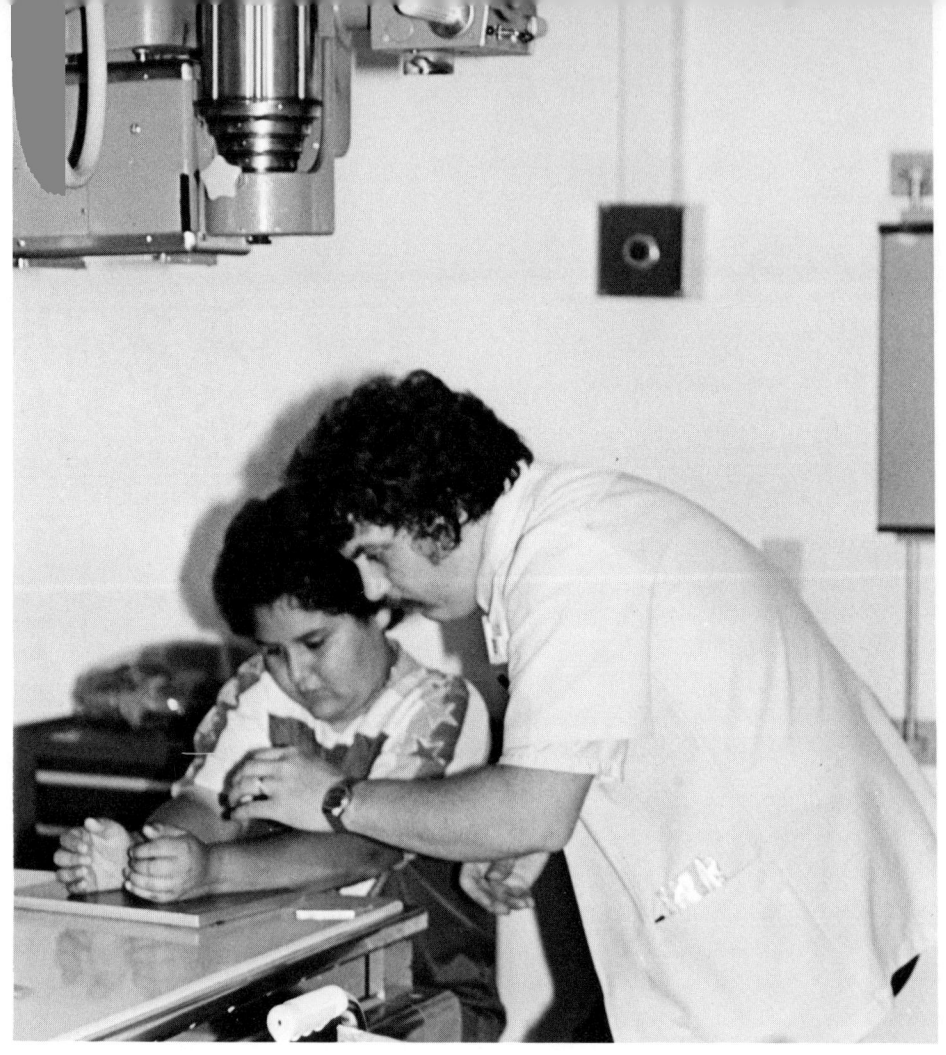

Health Care People

Nobody likes to be sick. Many people in the community work to keep us healthy. Health care people help to prevent sickness. They help to cure sickness. And they help us to feel better when we are sick.

Who are the health care people in your community?

Doctors and nurses are health care people. They know how to keep our bodies in good working order. They also know ways to help fix them when they are not working well.

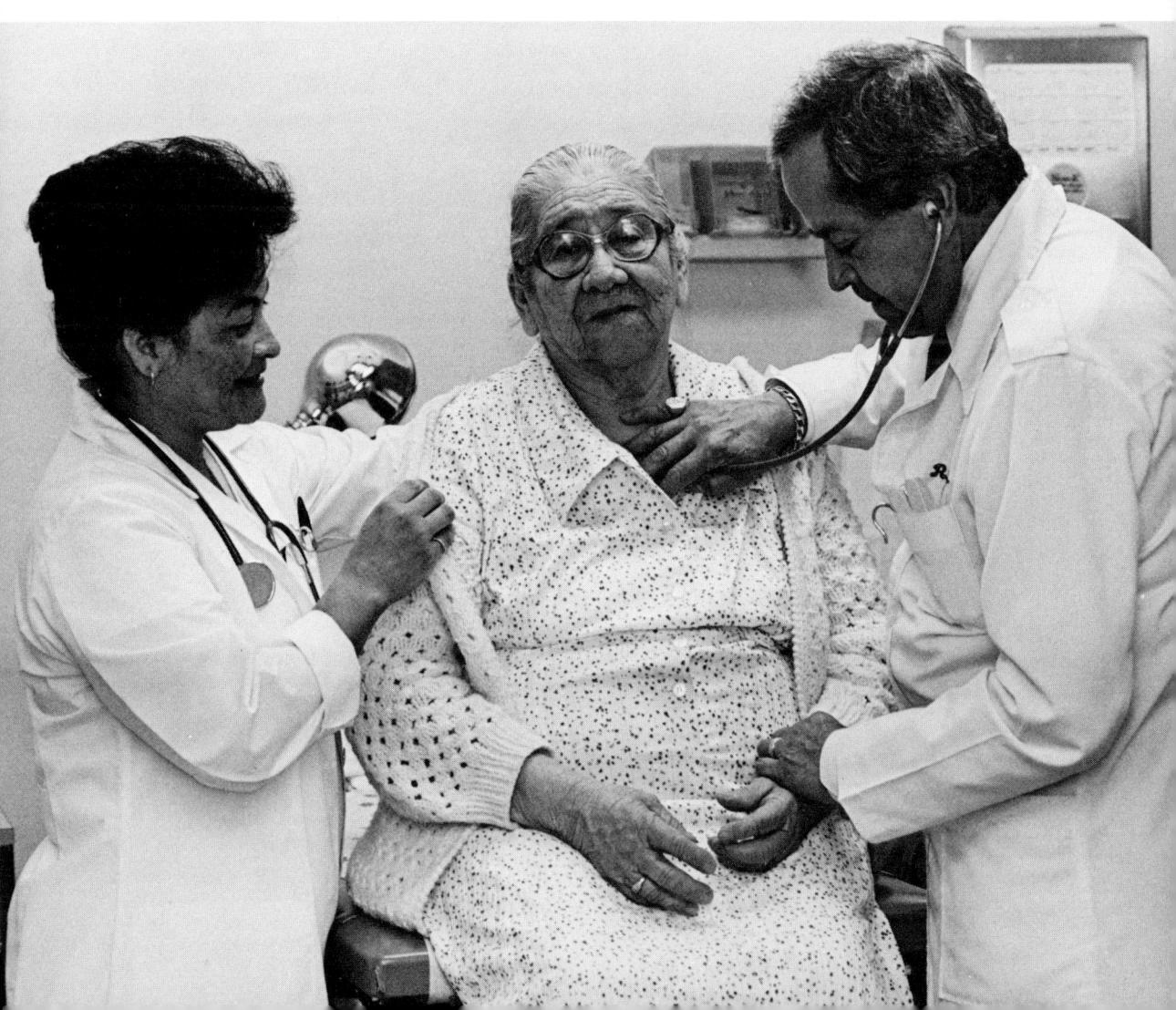

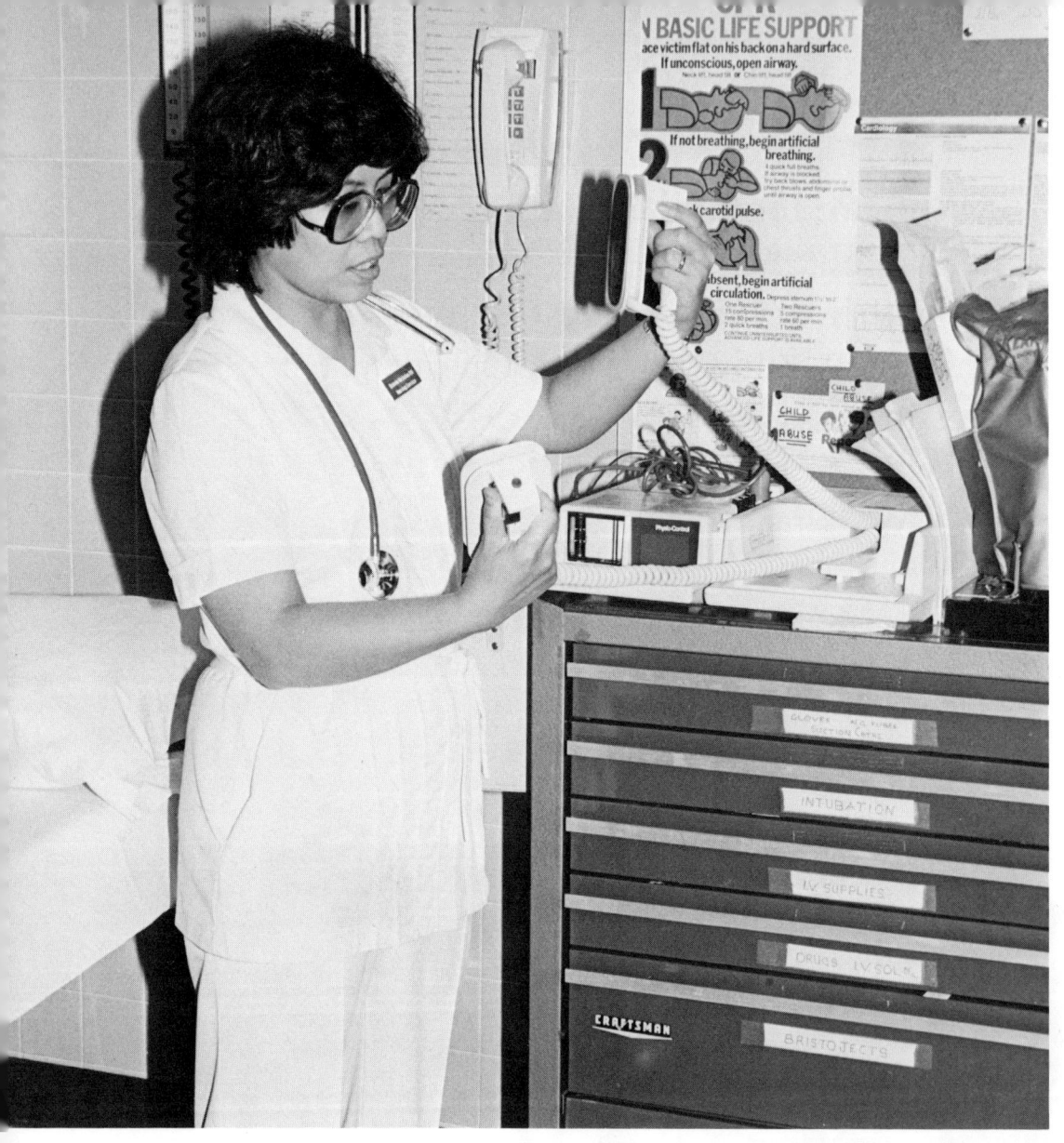

You go to a doctor when you feel sick or when you are hurt. The doctor will check you. Often a nurse helps the doctor. They will tell you what to do to get better.

There are many kinds of doctors. Some are eye doctors, foot doctors, and doctors that deliver babies. Doctors who take care of children are called pediatricians.

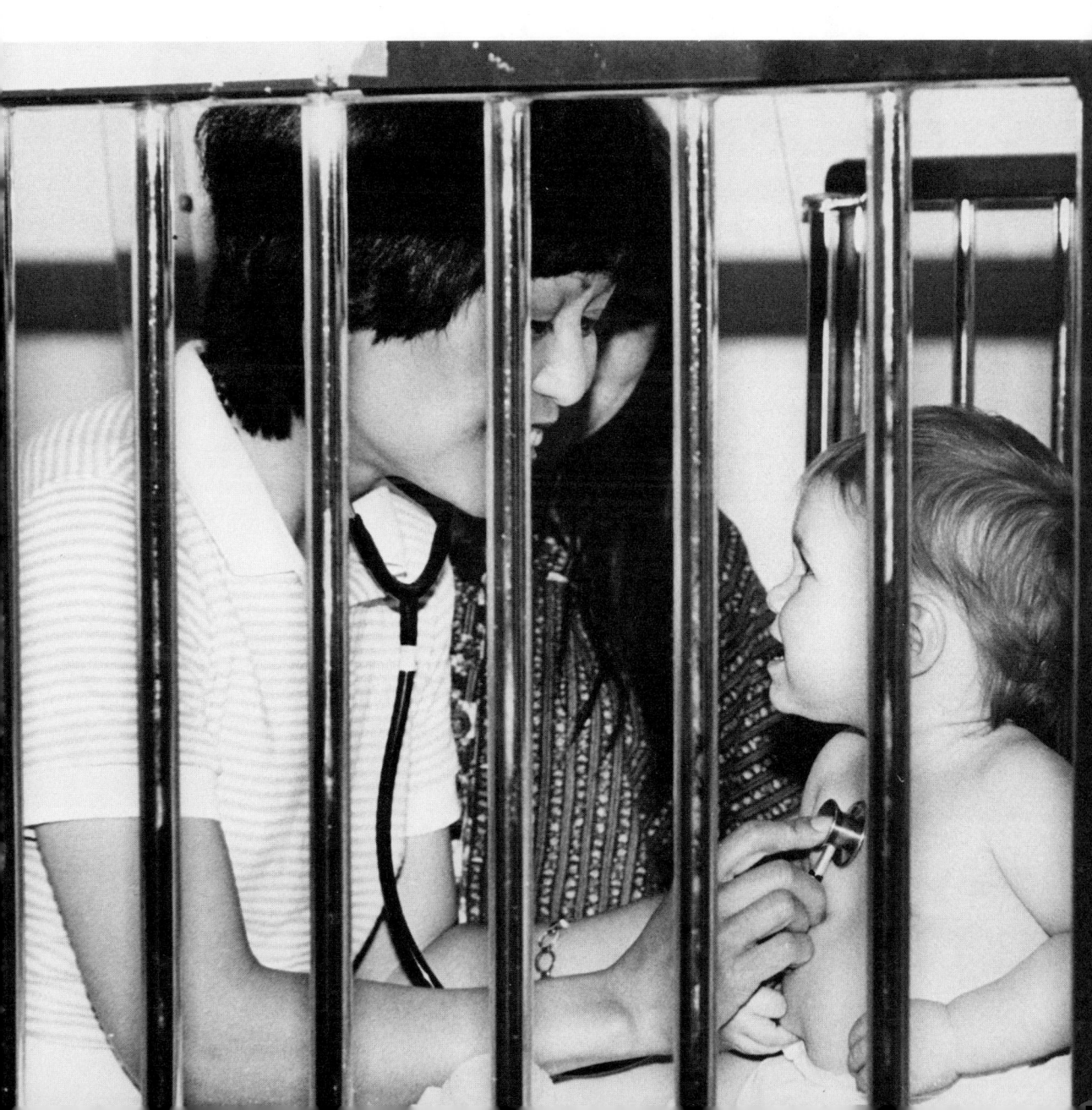

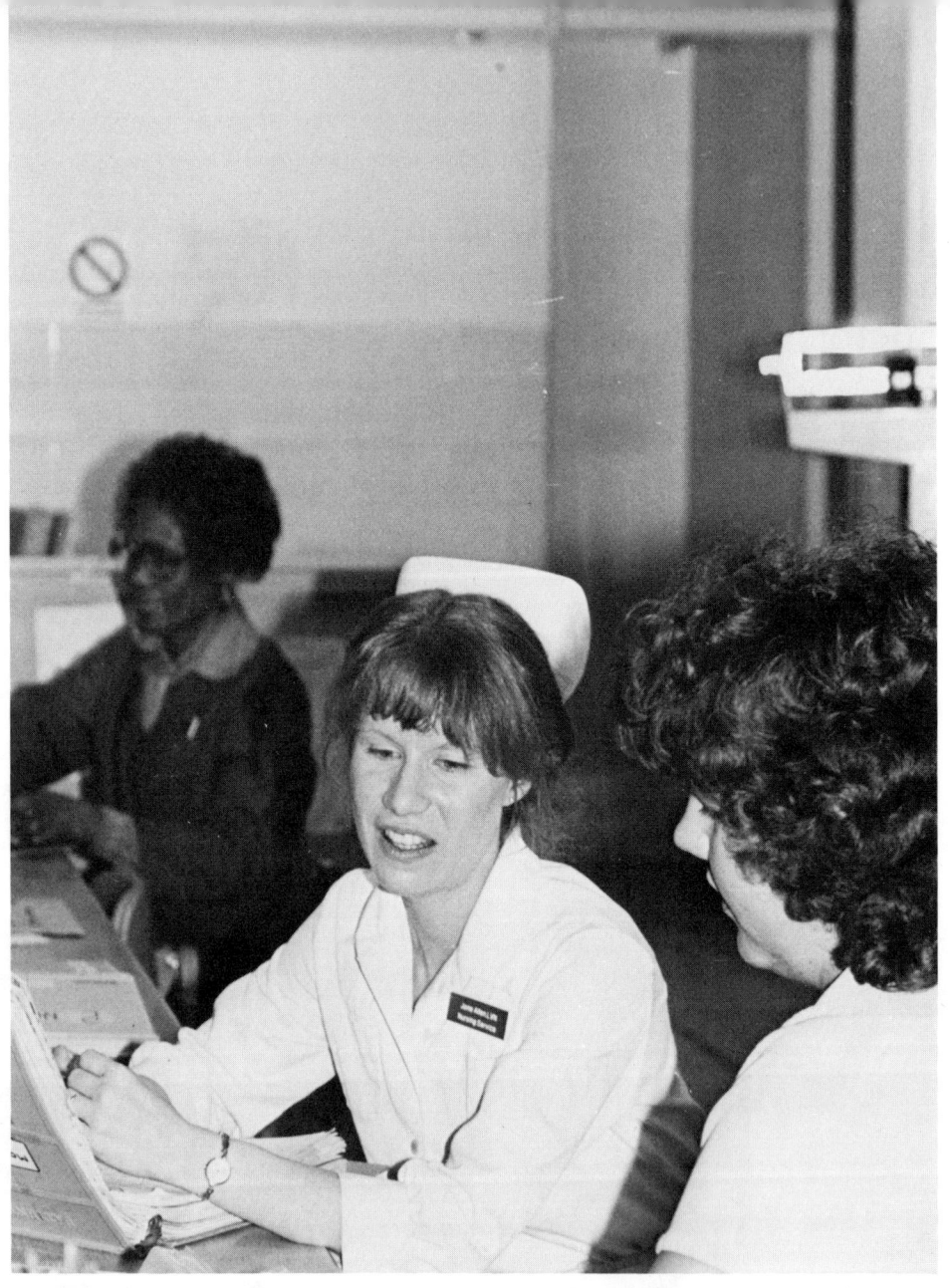

There are also many kinds of nurses. Some nurses work in doctors' offices. Some work in hospitals. Some nurses care for sick people at home. Many schools have a school nurse.

Sometimes you need medicine to help you get better when you are sick. Your doctor will write the name of the medicine on a piece of paper. This is a prescription.

Then you take the prescription to a drugstore. The druggist will sell you the right medicine. A druggist is also called a pharmacist. Pharmacists know about medicines and how to make them.

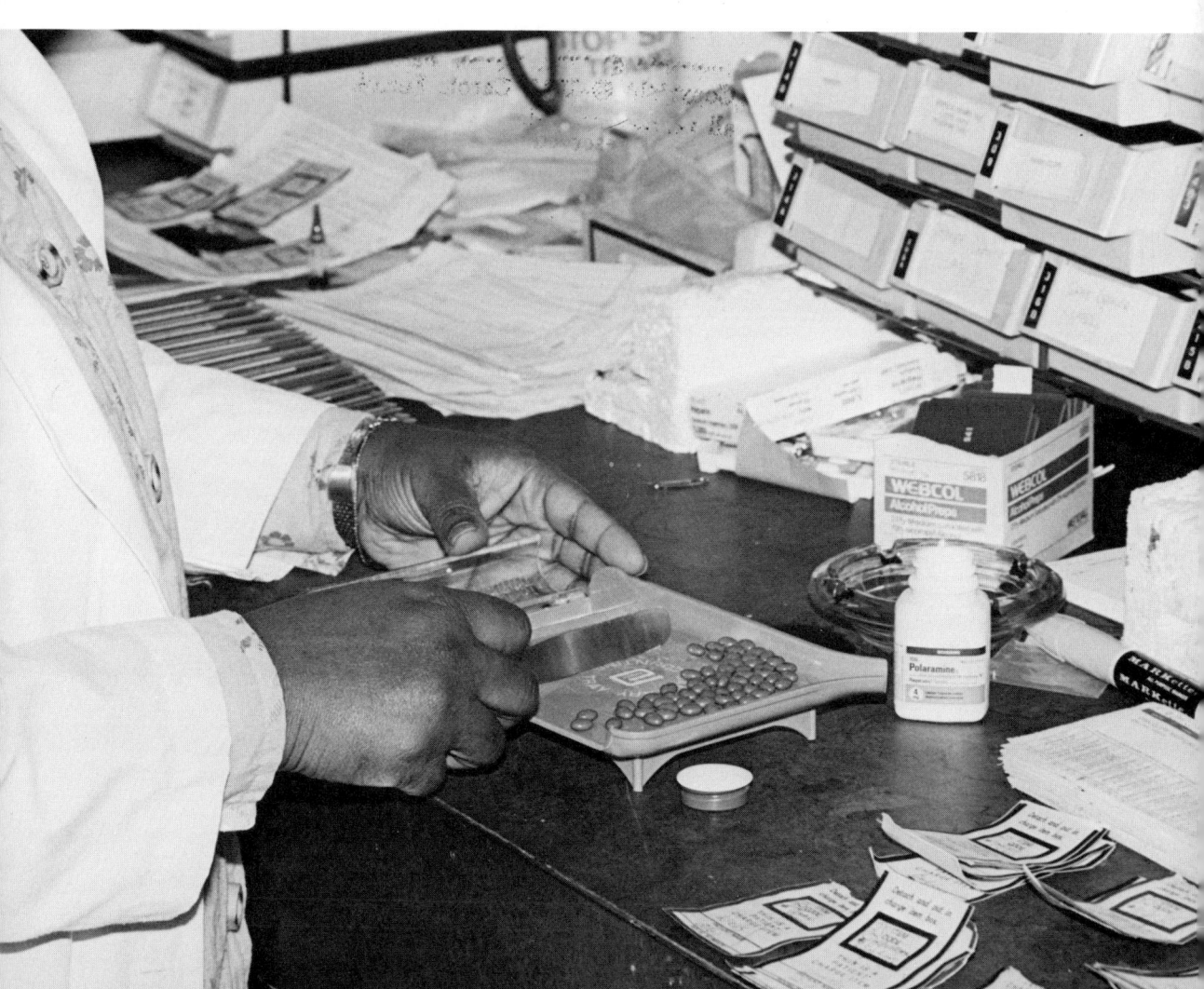

Dentists help you keep your teeth healthy. Most dentists have helpers. They are called dental assistants.

The dentist checks your teeth once or twice a year. He uses special tools to look at your teeth. He may also take X-ray pictures of your teeth.

Healthy teeth help us to bite and chew our food. You can help keep your teeth healthy. Eat good foods and brush each day.

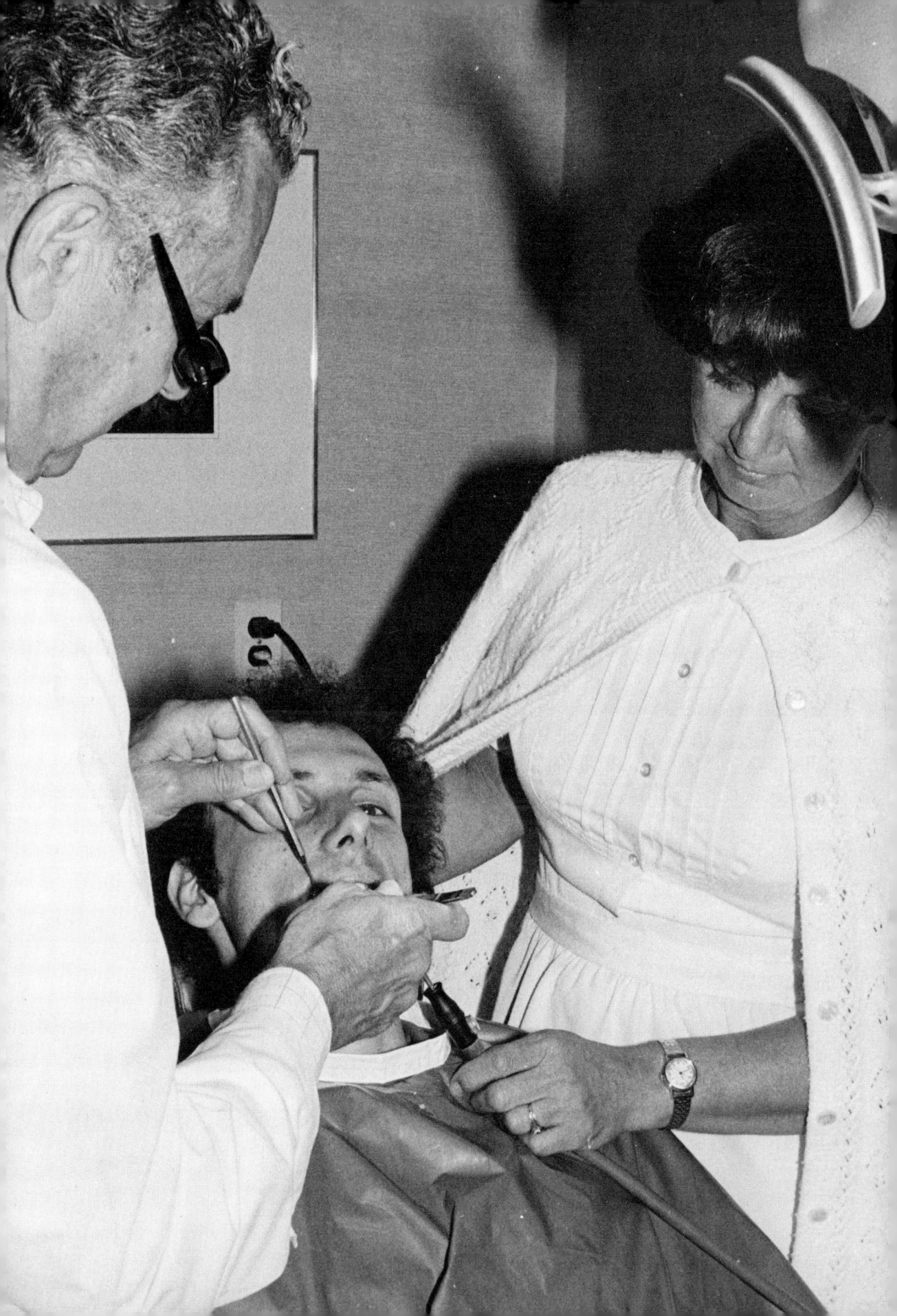

Do you have a pet? Sometimes your pet needs a checkup. Sometimes it gets sick. Then you need to take it to an animal doctor.

Animal doctors are called veterinarians or vets. Vets know how to take care of all kinds of animals. Some vets work in zoos. Others work with farm animals. Animals need to stay healthy just as people do.

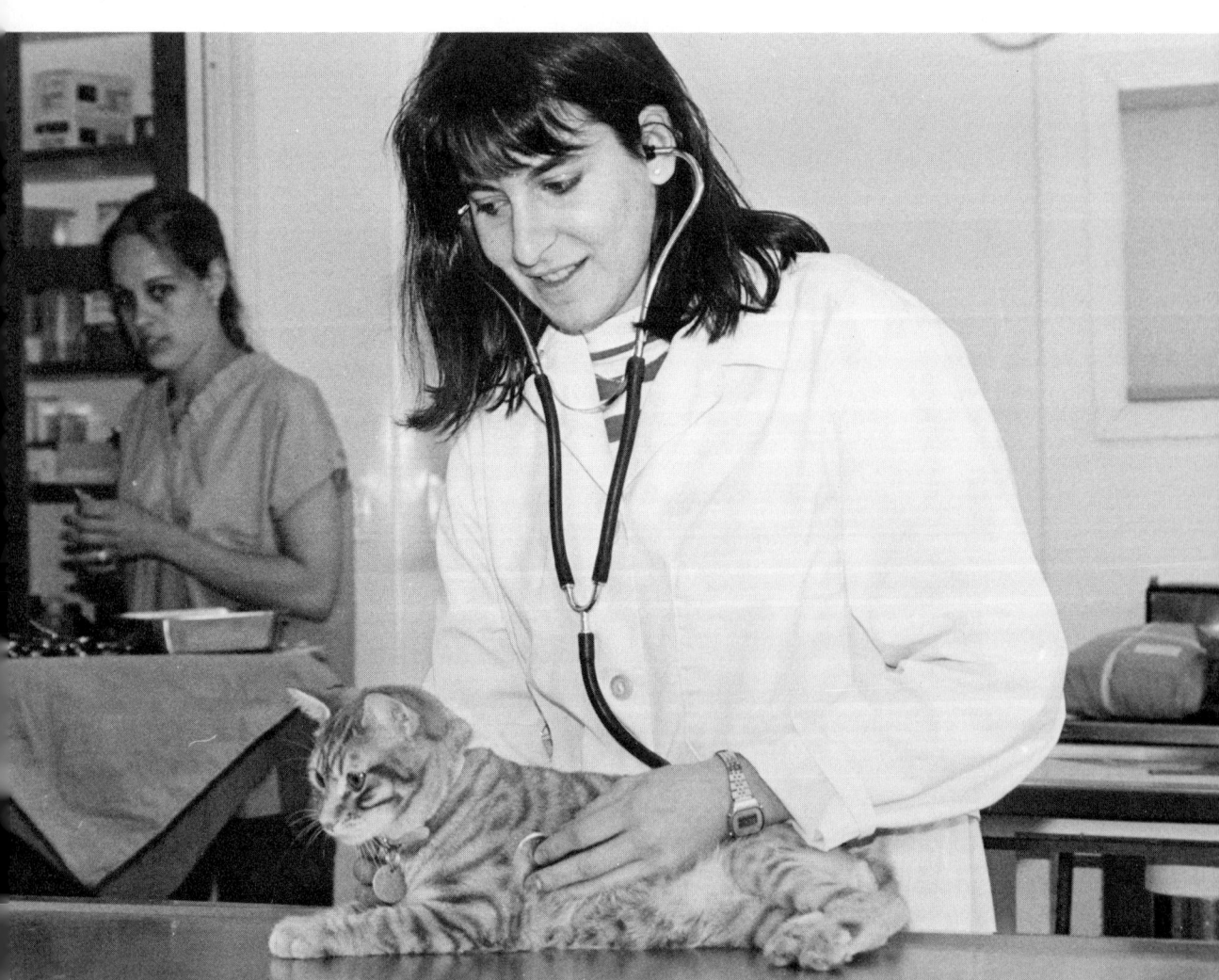

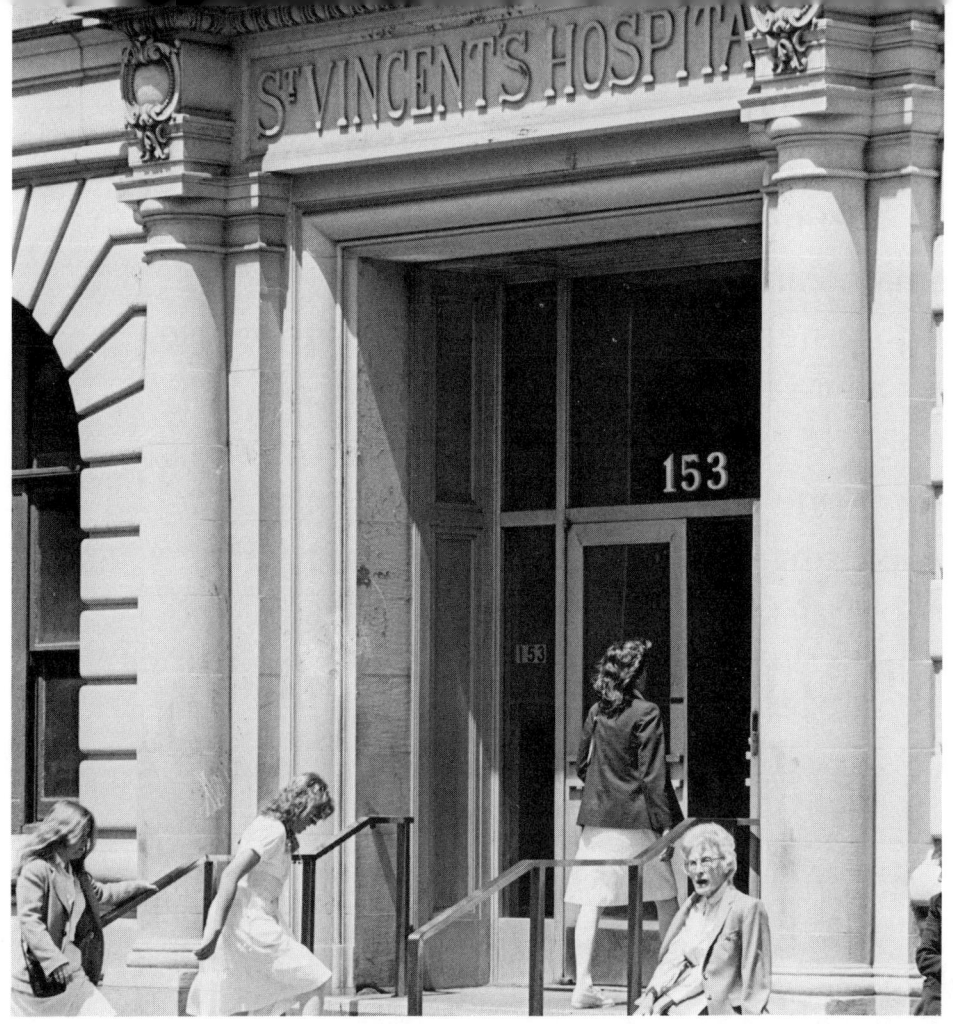

Places Where Health Care People Work

Many years ago most doctors went to people's homes. Today a few doctors will visit you at home if you are sick. But usually you must go to the doctor's office.

The doctor can treat you for most things in his or her office. But sometimes you must go to a hospital.

Some hospitals are big. Some are small. All hospitals have special equipment for doctors and nurses to use.

The emergency room is where people go who need care right away. If someone has an accident the ambulance will bring him or her to the emergency room as fast as it can. There doctors and nurses will be ready to help.

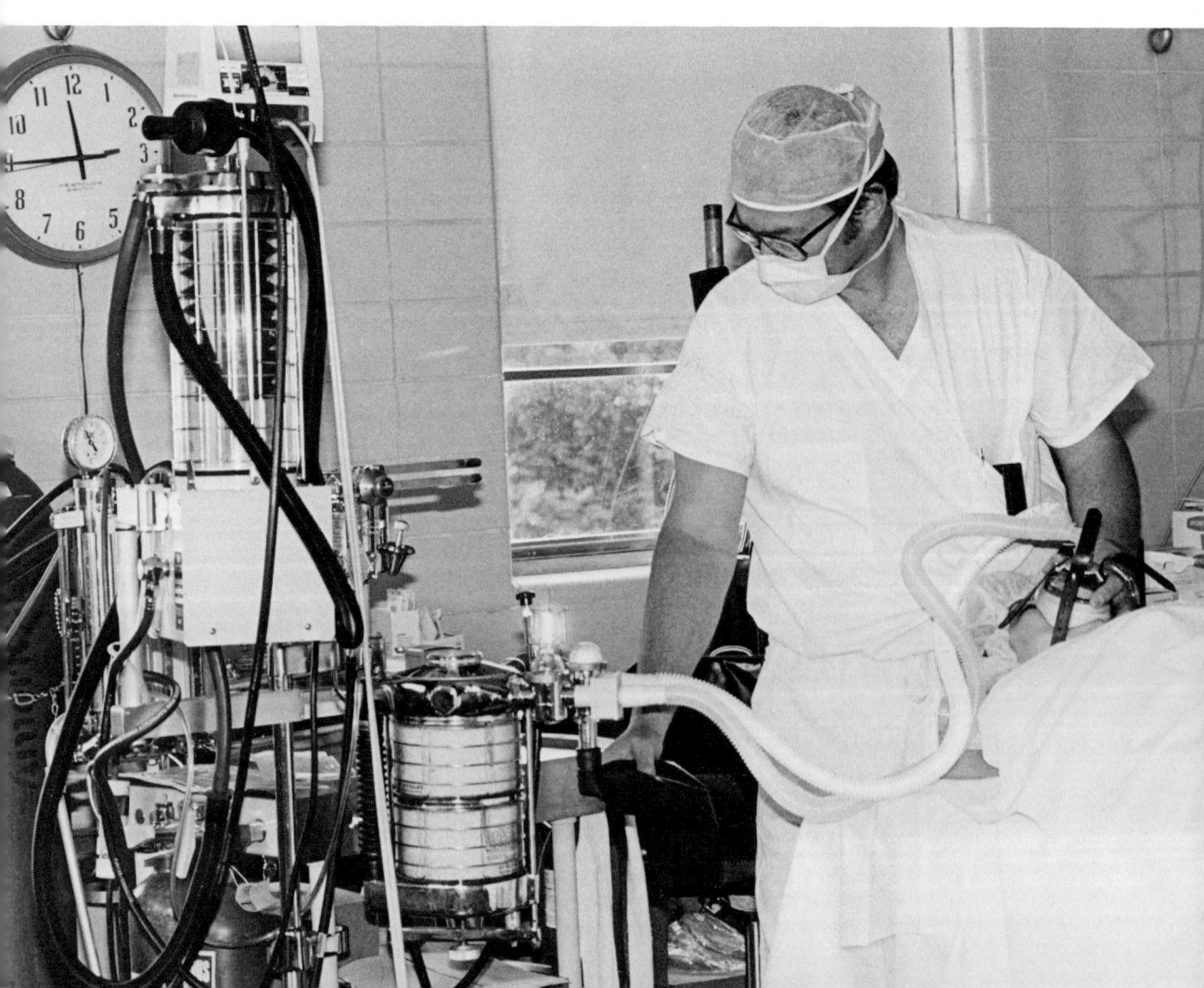

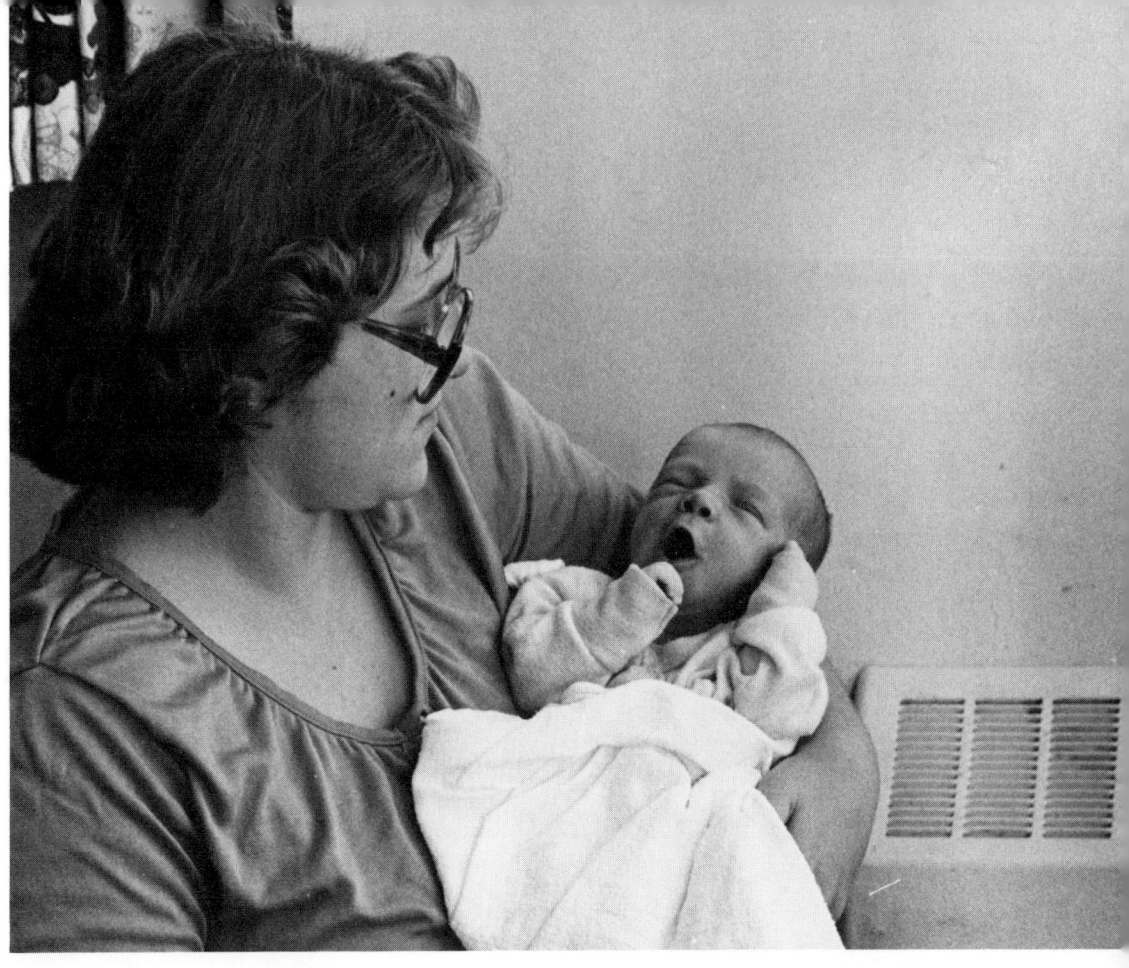

People go to hospitals if they are very sick. They also go if they get hurt badly. Sometimes people go to have an operation. Most mothers go to hospitals to have their babies.

Hospitals have beds for people to sleep in.

People stay in hospitals until they are well enough to go home.

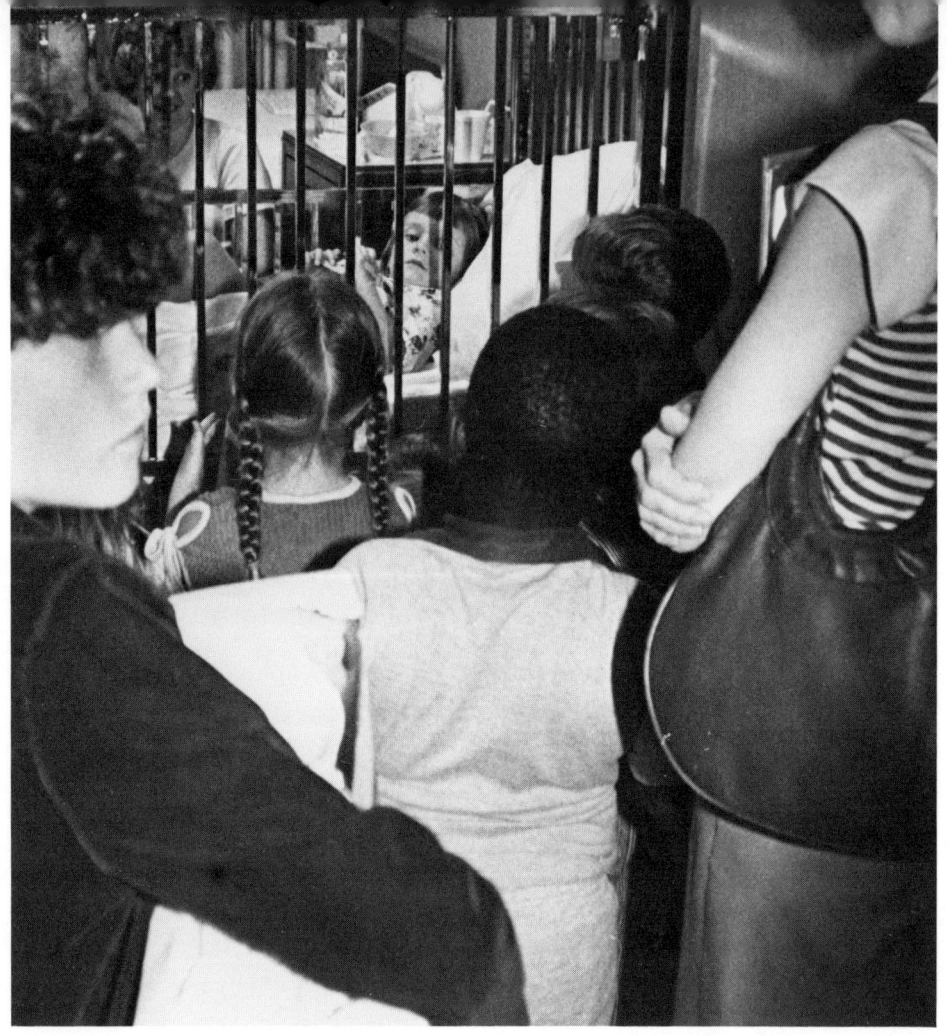

Hospitals have many rooms. Many hospitals have a part just for children. It may even have a playroom with toys. Everyone tries to make each child's stay as nice as possible.

Sometimes people have healthy bodies but unhealthy minds. Then they go to a psychiatric hospital. There doctors try to help them get better.

Many people work in hospitals.
Doctors and nurses give medical care. The dietician sees that everyone gets the right food. The physical therapist helps people do exercises to get better. The record librarian keeps all the medical charts in order.

Some people do medical tests. Many people keep the hospital clean. Hospitals bring together many kinds of health care workers.

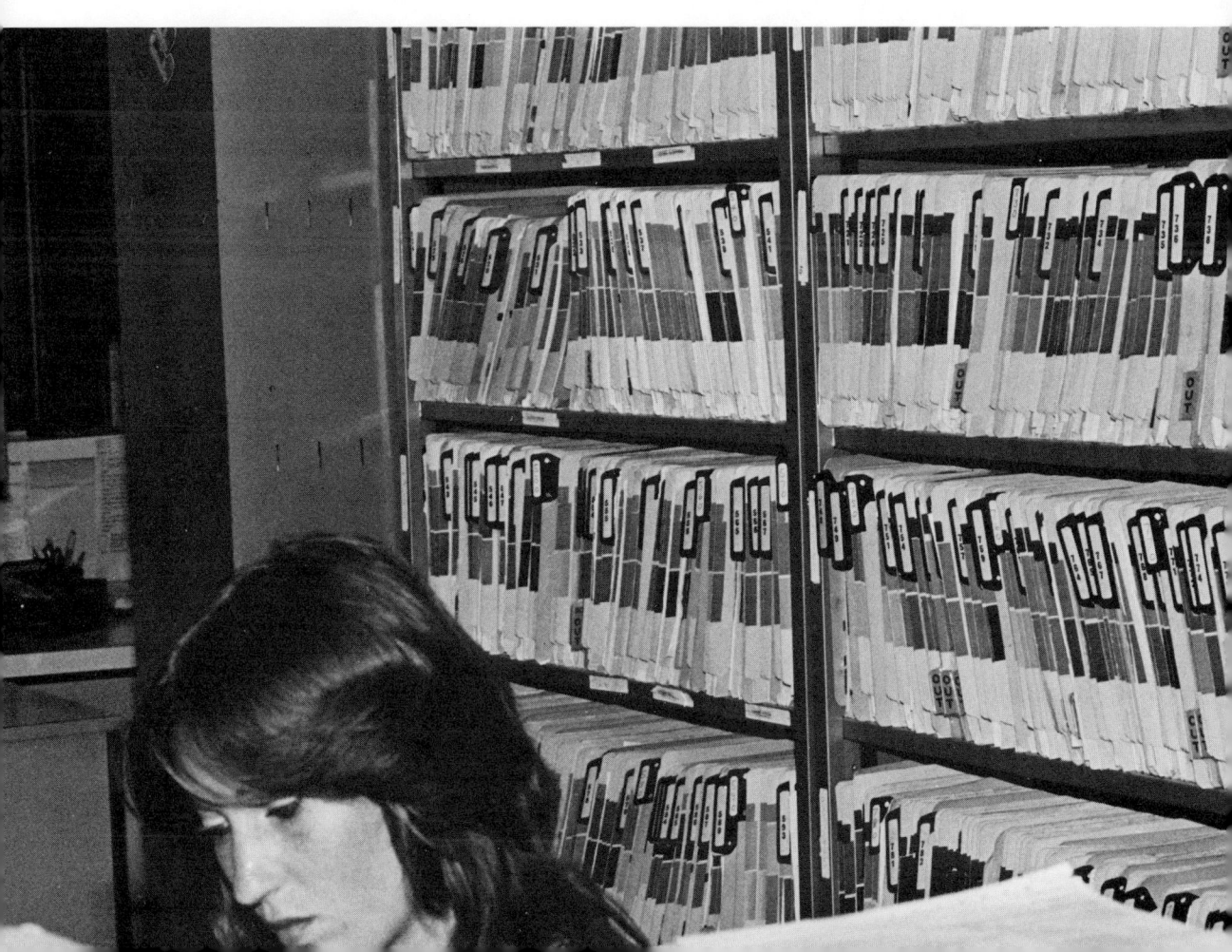

Old people are an important part of each community. Many communities have special places that care for old people.

Sometimes old people can no longer take care of themselves. Sometimes old people like to live near their friends.

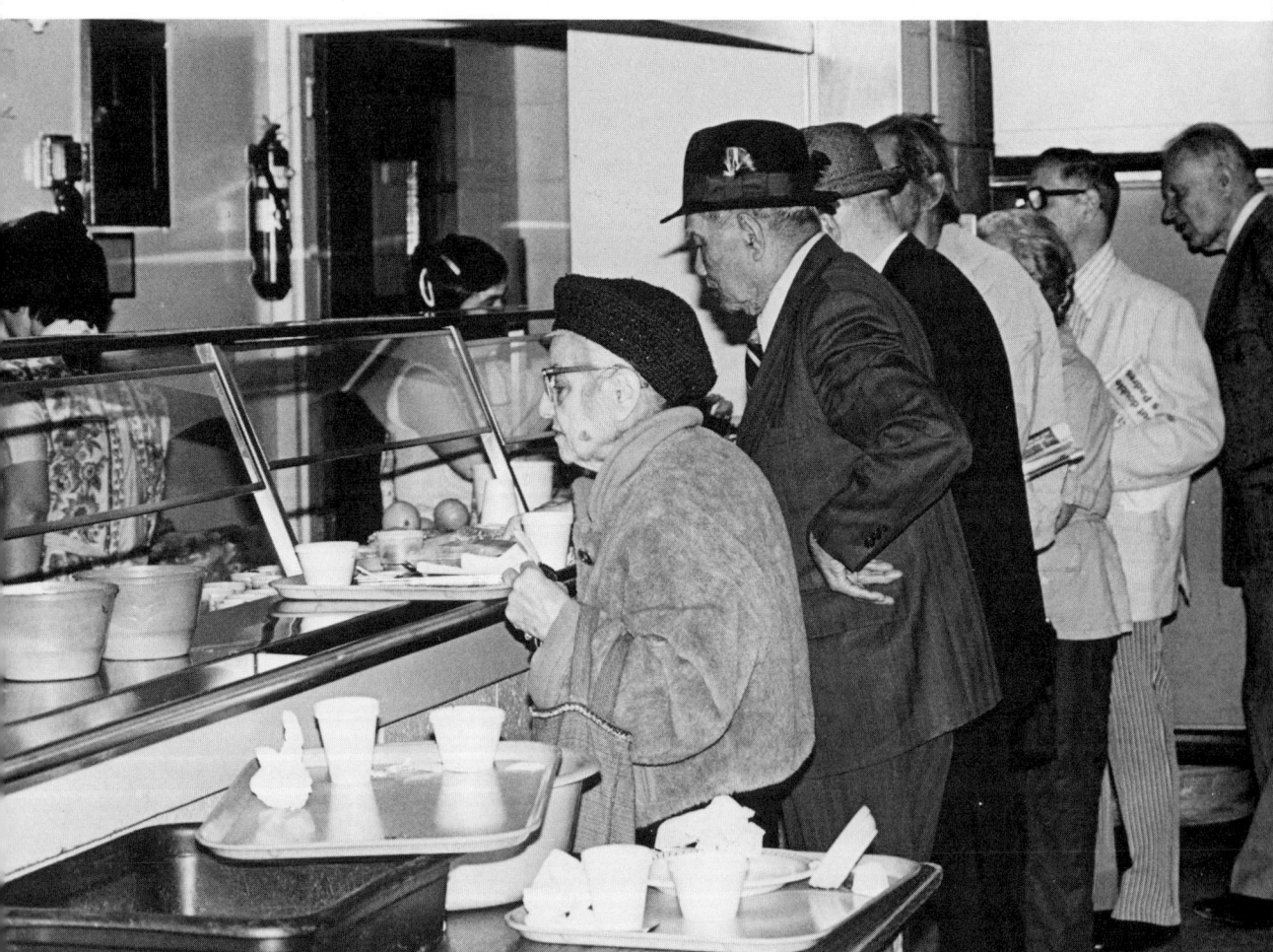

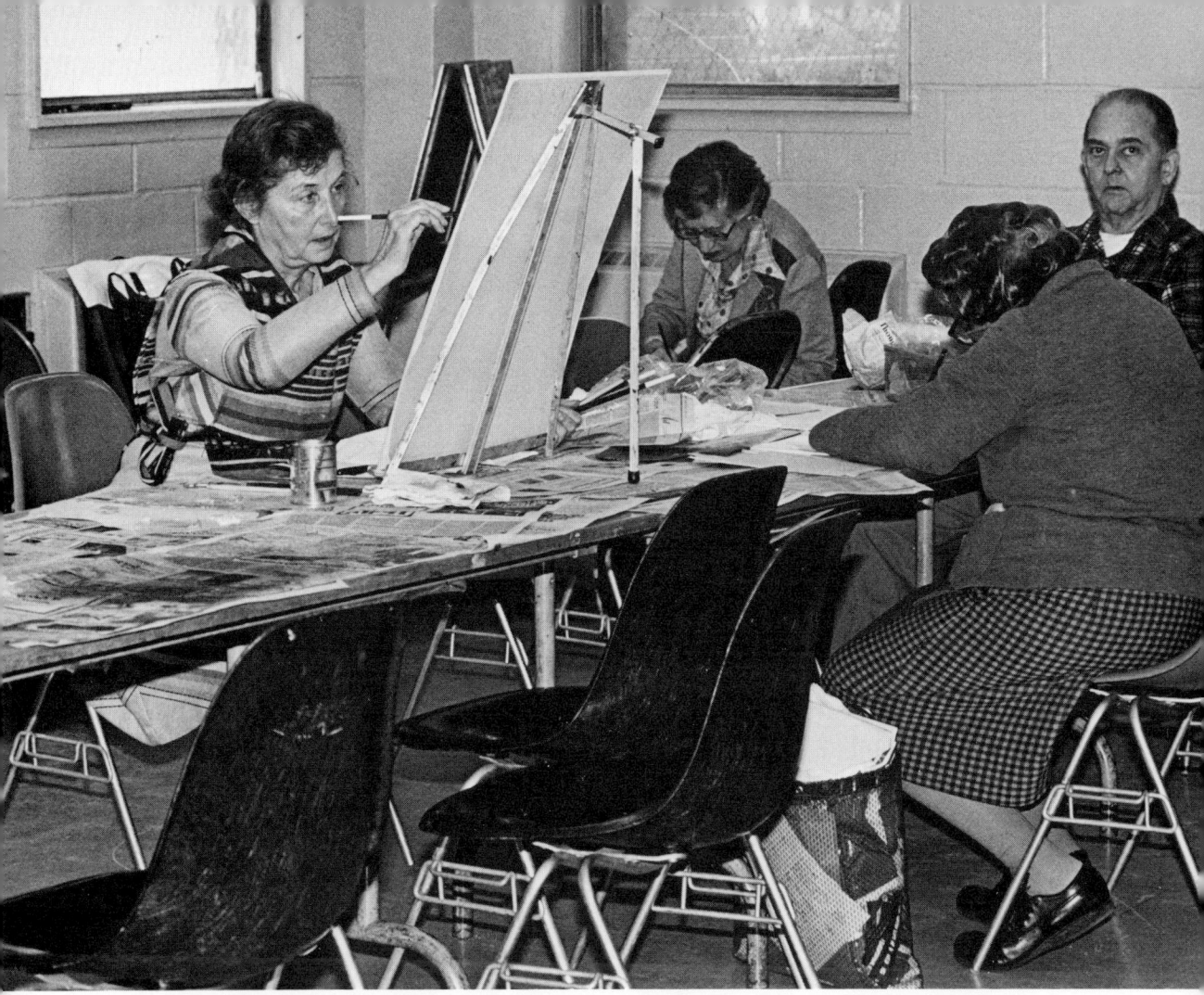

Homes for old people usually have nurses to care for people who are sick. They may also have dining rooms so people can eat together. They may have things for people to do.

In some communities people bring hot meals to old people who stay at home.

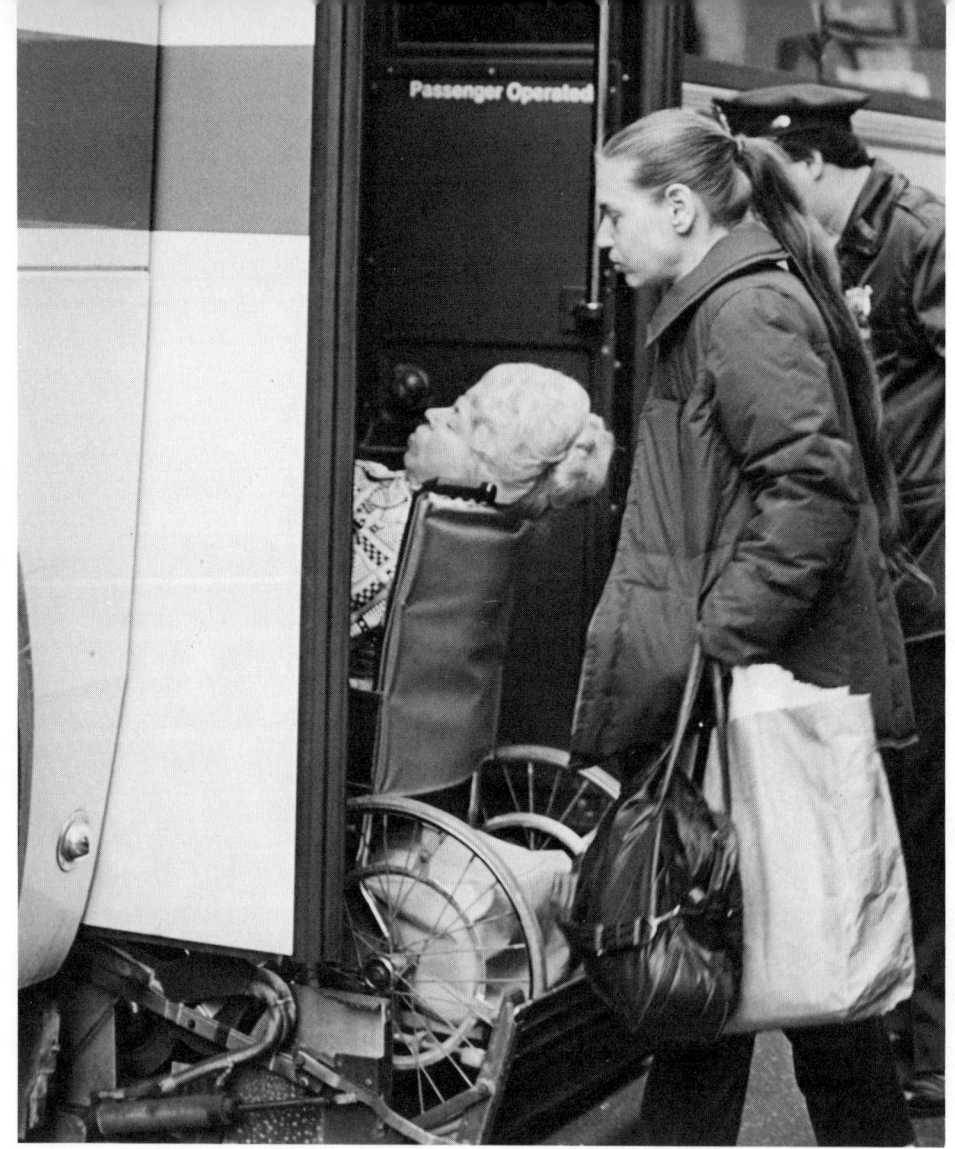

Many communities have special places for people with handicaps.

People who are blind or deaf may go to special schools.

People who use wheelchairs also need special care. Buildings must have ramps and wide doors for them.

People with learning problems need special care, too. Most people who have learning problems can learn to do certain things.

It is not easy to have a handicap. With help most handicapped people can have happy lives.

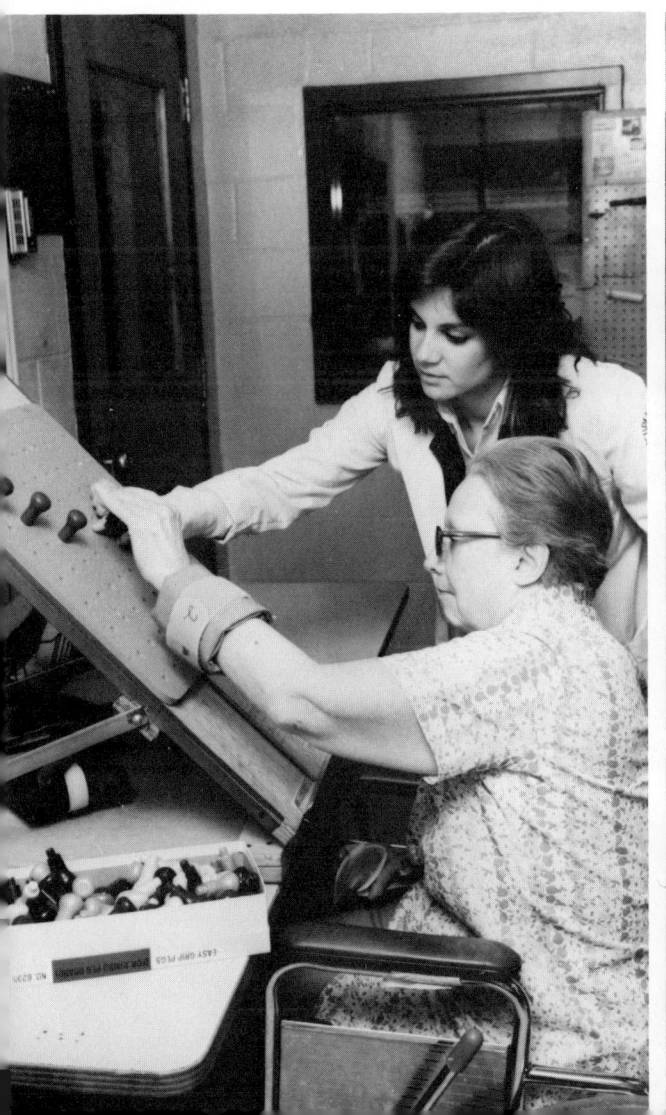
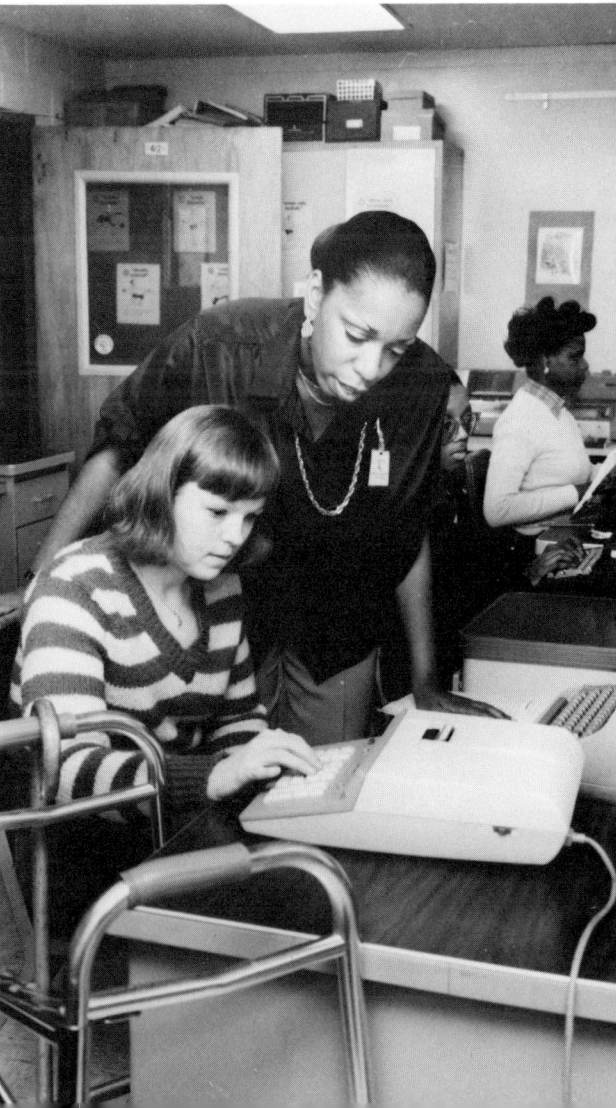

Communities Help People Stay Healthy

Many people work for good health in the community.

Some groups collect money. They use the money to help sick people.

Some groups teach us about good health. They teach about first aid and water safety. They teach parents how to take care of a new baby.

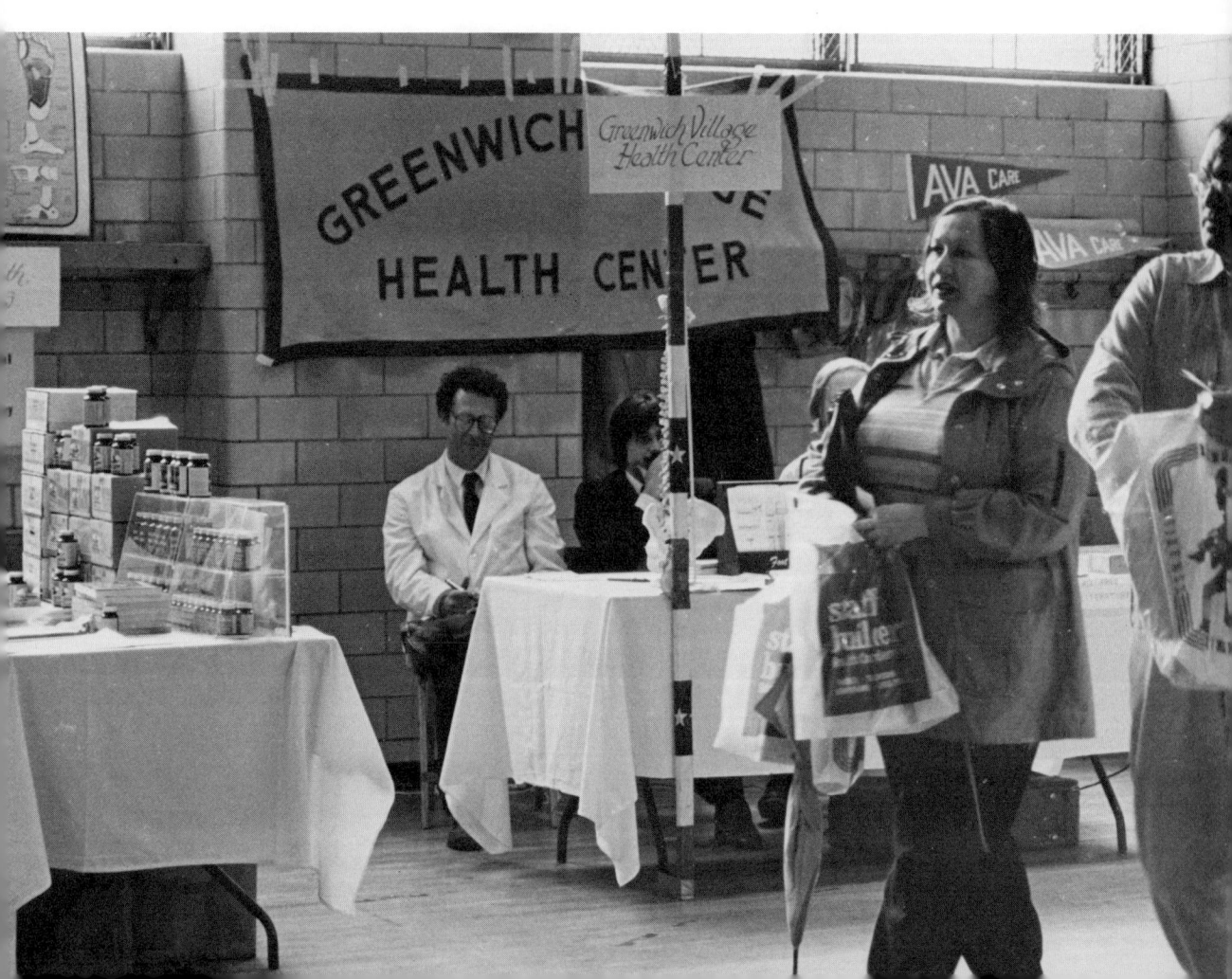

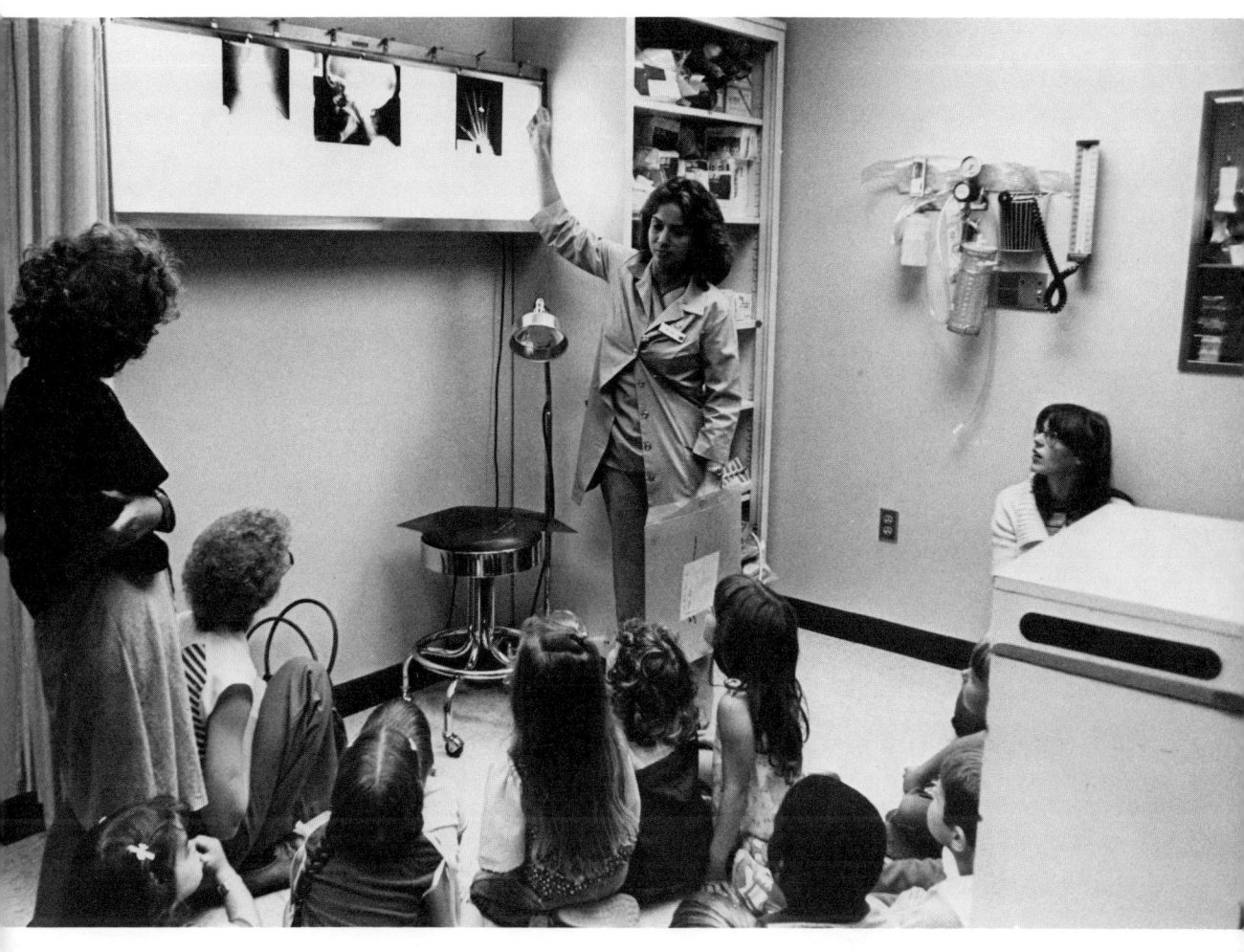

Some groups help people solve health problems. The problem may be drinking or smoking too much.

Some groups help people to get along better with each other. People are more healthy when they are happy.

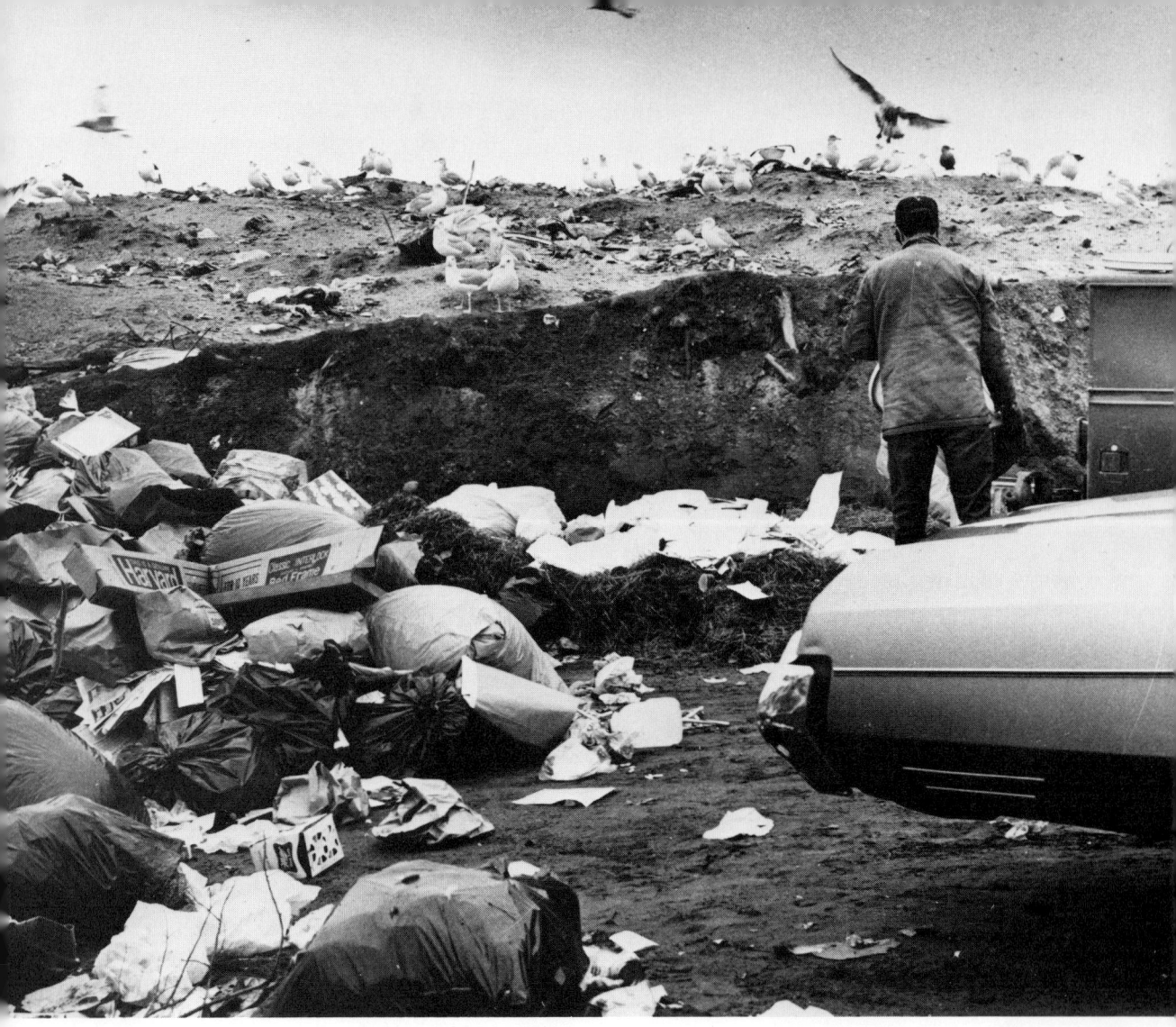

Germs make people sick. Germs grow and spread in dirty places.

Most cities collect garbage. They also have trucks that clean the streets.

In some communities each family must get rid of its own garbage. They may take it to a dump.

When the community is clean it is hard for germs to grow.

We all like to breathe fresh air. Communities try to prevent air pollution. Air pollution can make people sick. It may also smell bad and look bad.

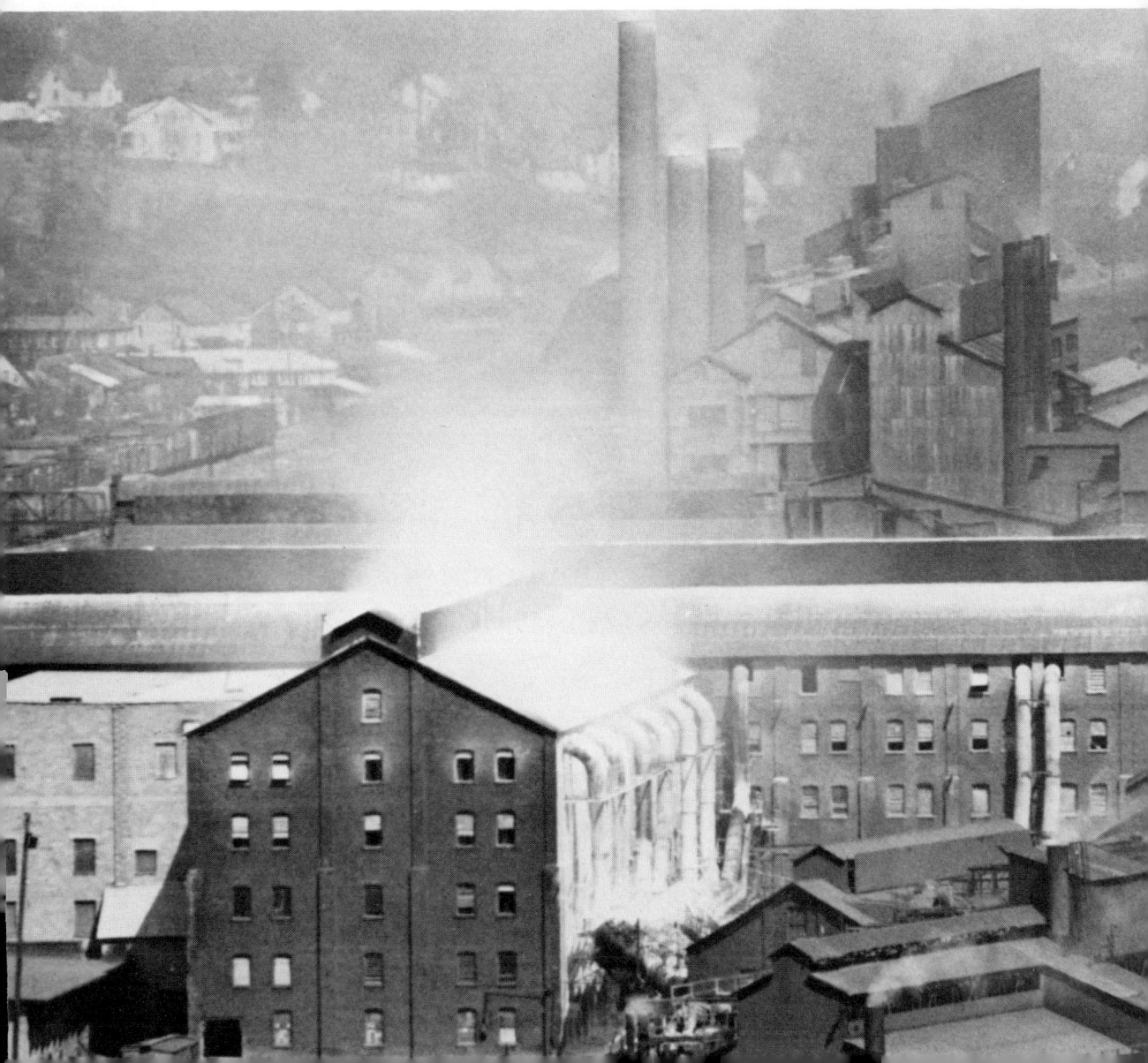

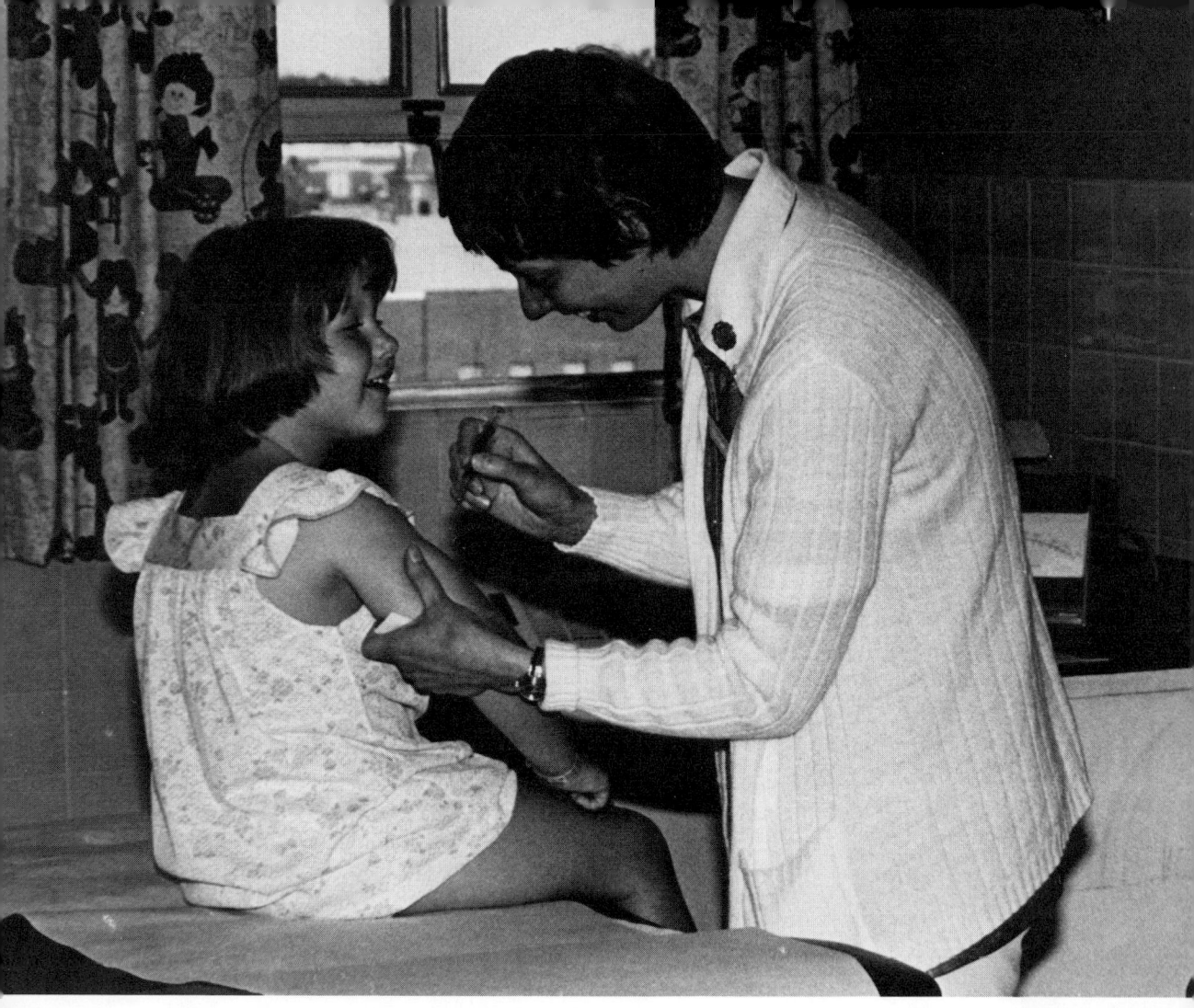

Many diseases can be prevented with vaccinations. In most communities children must have vaccinations before they start school.

A vaccination may hurt a little bit. But it is good for you. Vaccinations prevent many bad diseases.

Most communities provide people with clean drinking water. Small amounts of chlorine are added to the water. Chlorine is not bad for people. And it kills dangerous germs.

Some communities also have fluoride in their water. Fluoride helps to prevent tooth decay.

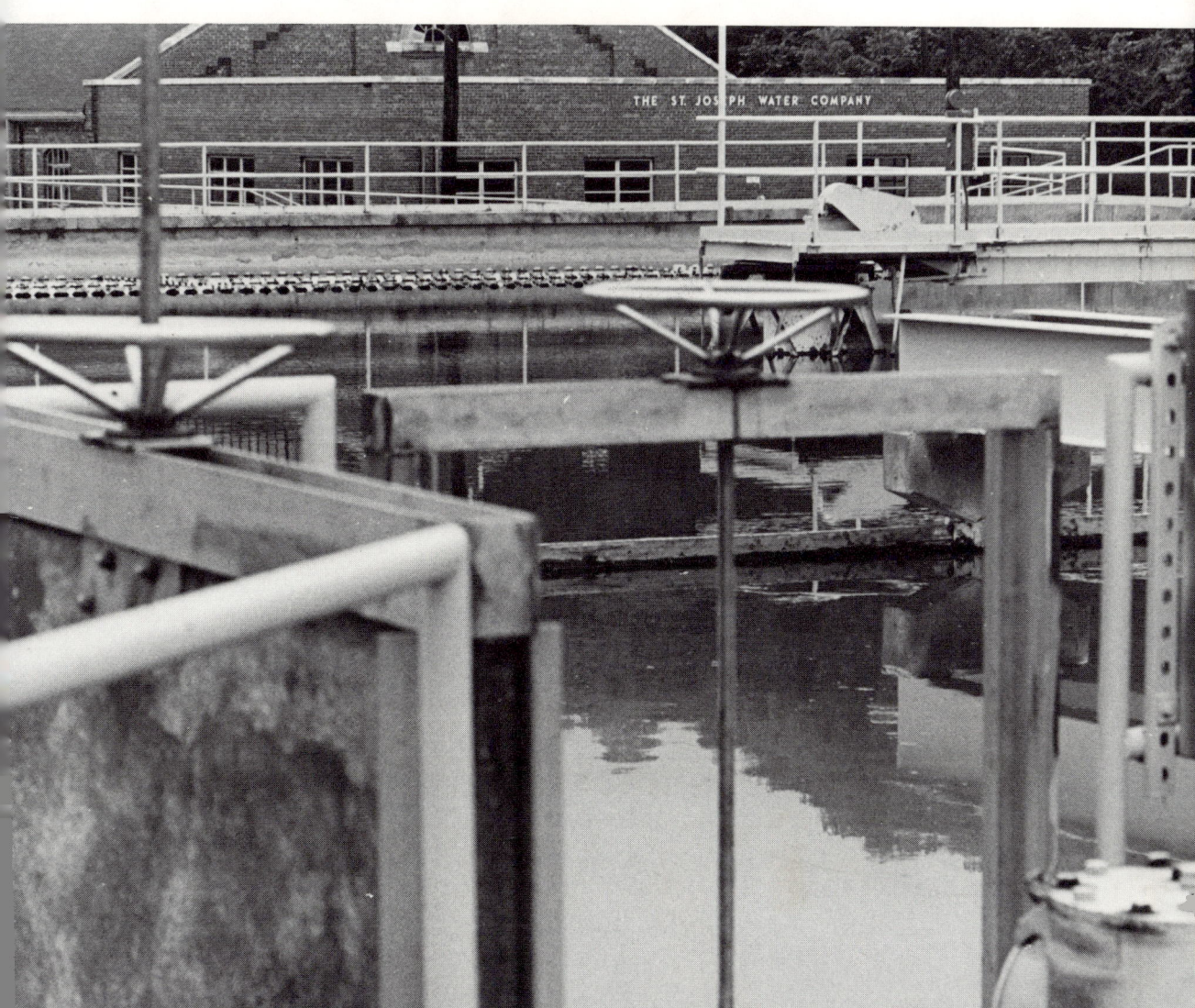

We all like to eat in restaurants. Most communities have people who check restaurants. They check the food to see that it is fresh. They check the kitchen to see that it is clean.

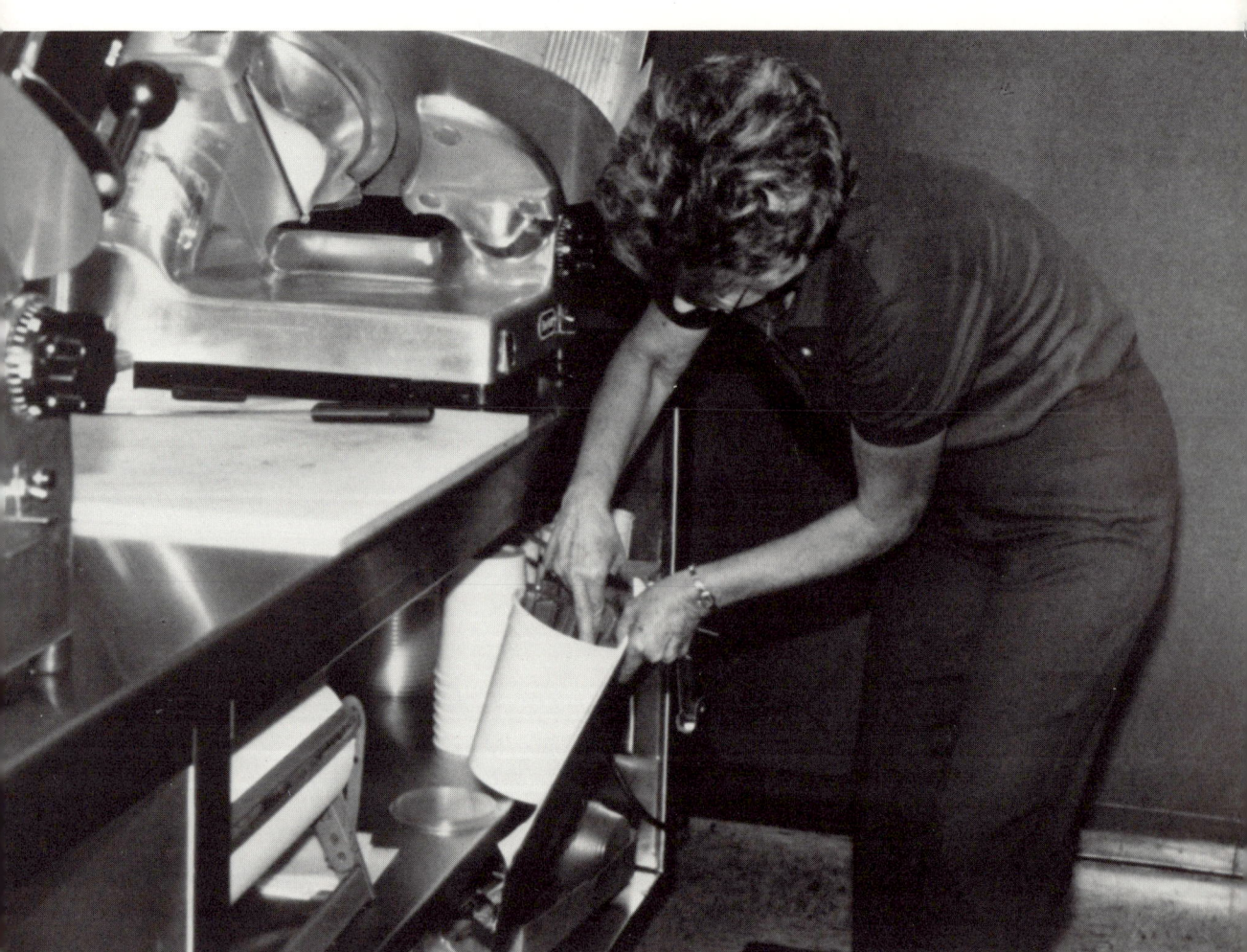

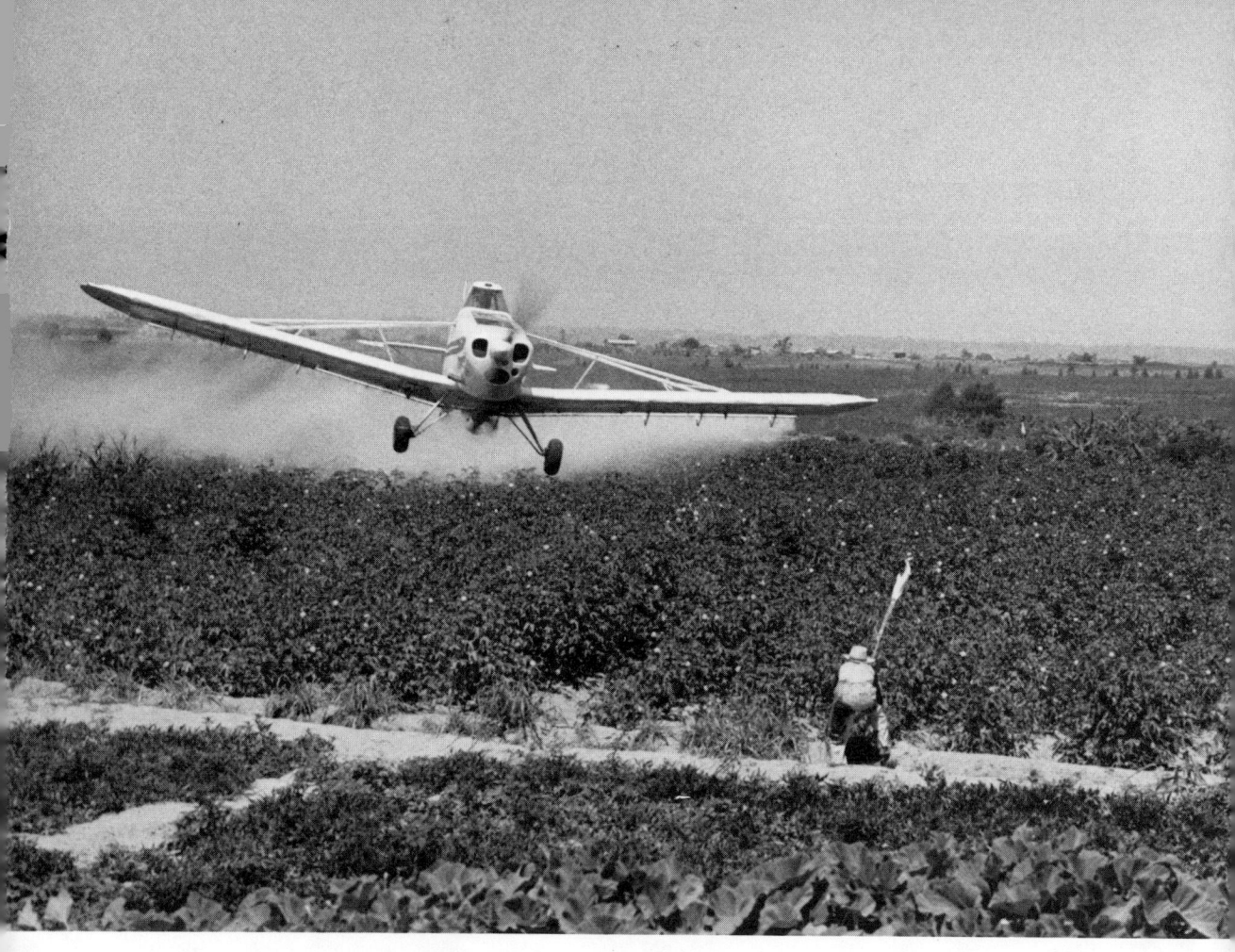

Some diseases are spread by insects. Many communities try to get rid of insects. They may drain swamps where insects grow. They may spray the insects with poison.

Animals like rats can also spread disease. Communities try to get rid of rats.

Good health is important for everything that people do. People cannot work or play when they are not healthy. In healthy communities people are happy.

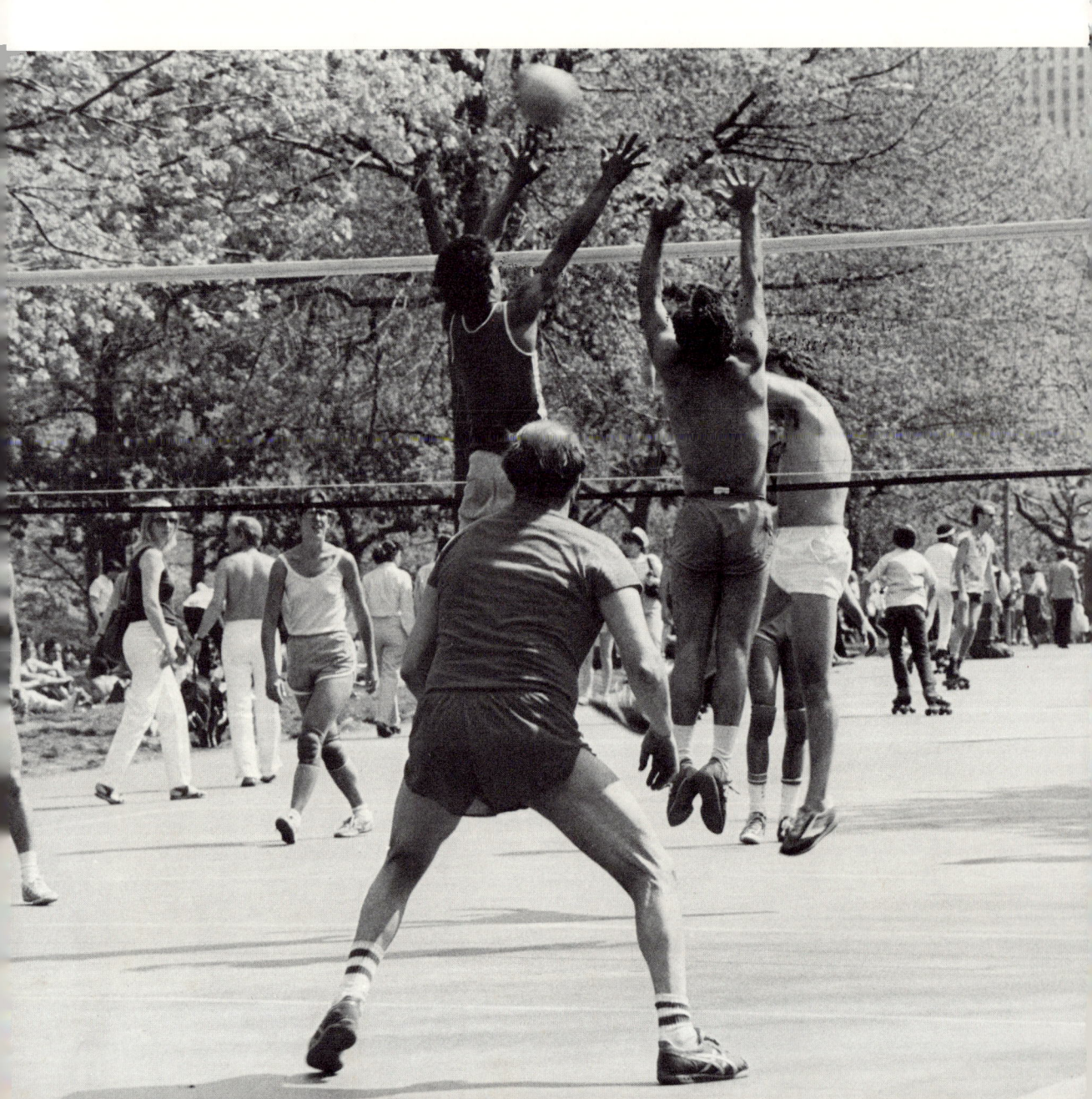